THE SILVER LINING
OF CANCER

13 Courageous Women Share Their Inspirational Stories
After a Life-Changing Diagnosis

TRACEY EHMAN

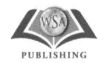

PUBLISHING

Published by
WSA Publishing
301 E 57th Street, 4th fl
New York, NY 10022

Manufactured in the United States of America, or in the United Kingdom when distributed elsewhere.

Ehman, Tracey
        The Silver Lining of Cancer: 13 Courageous Women Share Their Inspirational Stories After a Life-Changing Diagnosis

        LCCN: 2019902810
        Print: ISBN: 978-1-948181-53-2
        eBook: ISBN: 978-1-948181-54-9

Cover design by: Joe Potter
Copyediting: Claudia Volkman
Interior design: Claudia Volkman

 https://www.partneringinsuccess.com

Dedication

Dedicated to every person who has had cancer touch their lives.
Know that you are not alone.

Disclaimer

This book is not intended as a substitute for the medical advice of physicians. The reader should regularly consult a physician in matters relating to his/her health and particularly with respect to any symptoms that may require diagnosis or medical attention. The view expressed by each individual author are hers alone and not necessarily held by the other authors or by the publisher. Some names and identifying details have been changed to protect the privacy of individuals.

Table of Contents

FOREWORD

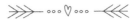

Gail Watson

I'm grateful to all the people in this book who had the courage and took the time to share their story.

Whether you are someone who currently is going through this disease, have come through it, or support and care for someone fighting it, we know that for many of us speaking our truth can be scary or even dangerous. Pain and suffering occur in silence, though, so when we can find our voice, we experience a newfound freedom.

I write this foreword as a close friend to the creator and lead author of this book, Tracey Ehman. I vividly remember the day when she shared with me those scariest words: "I have breast cancer." Silence and a sense of helplessness smothered me. Words ran through my mind—"What do I do? What do I say? How can I help? How do I just make this go away?"—but all that came out was "I'm sorry."

In her story Tracey shares the details of this time, including her extreme fear, anger, deep sadness, silence, strong determination . . . and then . . . the silver lining.

As she began to heal from the effects of chemotherapy, she shared those words with me and described what she called "the silver lining of cancer." I'm not sure if this disease transformed her or just brought out what was always inside of her, but during this time she saw the changes in her relationships with family, friends, business, life, and most importantly, herself. I witnessed her ease and peace as she appreciated the gift of time. She made time for people who were important to her. She made time for herself and scheduled in things that made her feel good. She had a newfound confidence and drive toward her abilities and her business. She inspired me through our daily conversations and taught me how to make "me time." She reminded me to not sweat the small stuff and to just breathe when things seemed to be out of control. The person who typically had played a support role to others was now the driver, leading the way.

This vision of this book was born during her journey. She wanted to share the stories of others who also saw and felt the silver lining. This book is for you.

If you are sitting in a medical waiting room right now waiting for treatment, may these stories give you strength, encouragement, and belief to know you have everything you need to get through this.

If you have just been diagnosed and heard the words "you have cancer" for the first time, may these stories provide comfort, give you hope, and let you know that you are not alone.

If you are supporting a family member or close friend who has been diagnosed and you are doing your best to stay strong and offer the right words to them, allow these stories to remove the fear and guide and inspire your words and actions.

It took great courage and vulnerability for each author to share her deeply personal experience. The stories and emotions in this book are raw and real, and they freely shared to give you, the reader, hope, inspiration, support, and love.

You are not alone.

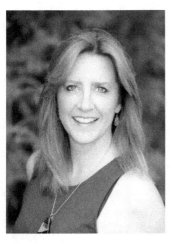

GAIL WATSON *is president and founder of Women Speakers Association (WSA), the go-to place for innovative leaders, change-agents, and women with a message to connect, collaborate, and grow their visibility worldwide in order to fulfill their mission. As the first-ever global community for women speakers, WSA provides a platform for women to get seen, booked, and paid AND be part of a growing network reaching women in 120 countries.*

www.womenspeakersassociation.com

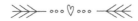

I don't know exactly what the future holds,
but I'm stepping forward with grit and grace.

JOHN GRAHAM

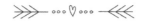

EVERY EXPERIENCE YOU HAVE SHAPES YOUR FUTURE

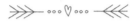

Tracey Ehman

While I wouldn't wish cancer—or any illness, for that matter—on anyone, I do know that in my case, it helped shape who I have become. Not the disease itself so much, but the ability to find gratitude in the positives and take advantage of opportunities that have come my way because of it. In fact, the birth of *The Silver Lining of Cancer* was a result of conversations I had with a good friend, about taking what I had experienced and overcome to inspire others. I didn't know at that time what it would look like, but ultimately, when this option was presented to me, I knew it was the perfect platform to help inspire, provide hope, and share that others have walked the same path. While the journey is not a pleasant or positive one for many, being able to be in gratitude and find the silver lining can make the journey more bearable.

I grew up in the Vancouver area with my mom, dad and sister. Family was and always has been an important part of our lives—church on Sunday, breakfast with cousins afterward, amazing dinners with my grandparents on both sides. I loved that I had my grandparents around for a long time growing up.

1

The year following my wedding, my mom called me to let me know that she had found a lump that had been confirmed to be cancer. At the time, I was taking three classes a semester as well as working full-time. I remember taking an exam the night after I found out. It was incredibly hard to concentrate, and it was probably my worse test score ever, but my thoughts were focused on my mom. It was so scary for me, as her daughter—wondering what I could do, thinking about what might happen if things didn't go well. . . . It still makes me so emotional when I relive that time. But Mom was a trooper—and you can read her story in this book too.

Flash forward seventeen years later. I had begun to create a good business, including virtual assistance and website and social media management, and was feeling more and more confident that I could build it big. I was working a ton of hours, and not eating well—in fact, my staple began to be soy nutritional bars for breakfast and lunch. I had gone for a mammogram in February, something I did earlier because of the potential for me to also be predisposed to breast cancer. All was good. But a month later, I felt a lump. I don't know when it appeared, but I knew it wasn't there the month before, so I hoped it was related to something more hormonal. But when you know, you know. You don't really need someone to tell you that you have cancer . . . but that confirmation makes it so real!

Within a month I had a needle biopsy, a breast MRI, and surgery. My doctor suggested that I think about a mastectomy, but it was important for me to fight to keep all that was mine, and that included my breast. I talked to the surgeon and he agreed that a lumpectomy (partial mastectomy) was the right choice. And he did an amazing job! One of the silver linings that I see now looking back was understanding the importance of self-advocacy. If something doesn't feel right, or you need more information, you need to speak up.

I remember people offering their opinions of what they would do if they were in my situation, and yet no one can really know what they will do until they have to make those decisions for real. I know people were trying to be helpful, and giving me advice was a way to share their love. I chose to go for chemo and radiation, as I wanted to be sure that I annihilated those nasty cells. It was my choice, and I stand by it today.

During this time my daughter turned fourteen and my son was ten. I knew I had to be strong for them, especially having been in their shoes so many years before. My husband, children, family, and friends were my source of normalcy, and I appreciated all of them more than I can adequately express. My husband taught me to not concentrate on the "what ifs" and instead deal with things as they came. I truly believe that this experience taught my children empathy, sympathy, love, gratitude, and the power of choosing to see the glass as always half full. There were tough times, but we came out the other side stronger.

For me, what really worked was being able to concentrate on working for my clients. I was able to channel my energy into growth, creation, and success rather that dwell on being sick. I was rarely sick before, so having my body dictate what I could and couldn't do was something I couldn't allow. I believe communication is always important in any aspect of your life, and I made sure to let my clients know when I would be having chemo treatments. I told them that I expected to be doing limited work for seventy-two hours afterward, so they would get anything that needed to be done to be prior to my treatment. This worked well. In fact, I actually tripled my business while going through treatment. It was empowering!

I continued to live my life while going through treatment and life-changing experiences along the way. I was determined not to miss out on anything. I even made it to the annual Christmas party I had attended for twenty-two years, and I celebrated my last chemo treatment on December 29th at a New Year's party. I was determined to maintain my normal, even if it was a different version of normal. Complete with my new, lighter hairstyle, I maintained as much of a social life as I could. I found that it helped me more to be out with family and friends than to hide away like I wanted to do. Everyone is different in how they process info, deal with adversity, and find a way to get through whatever they need to overcome.

I am happy to be healthy and happy eight years later, and I always have felt that I wanted to make a difference. I know that I found inspiration and calmness by talking to others who had been through similar circumstances when I was going through my cancer journey. And it was important to me to share with others.

I am so honored to have these incredible women join me in sharing their stories and making an impact. The stories include a woman who overcame everything that was thrown at her to find her wings; a daughter who found the beauty in how her mother dealt with her illness and the wisdom she shared; a daughter, sister, and niece who saw her family being impacted by numerous cancer diagnoses and chose to embrace her own health; an entrepreneurial woman who knew that something just wasn't right and made changes by healing through love; a cancer thriver who recently lost her brother but still chooses to find the silver lining through her grief; a woman who realized that she needed to take stock of her life and make changes to reduce stress; a healer who turned her gifts into a golden elixir that helped her heal; a woman who realized it was OK to accept help; a breast cancer survivor who found the twelve blessings on her journey; and a woman who came back from a prognosis of brain cancer.

I'm sure you will find a chapter that speaks just to you. I'm hoping that this book helps you find *your* silver lining.

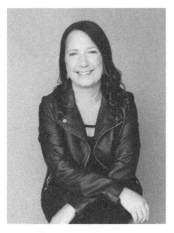

TRACEY EHMAN *is a wife, the mother of two, and a social media strategist who tripled her business while going through chemotherapy and radiation. Because of her ability to concentrate on the positive, even in adversity, she was driven to share her story and provide a vehicle to help others also share their stories and inspire people to always look for the silver lining.*

www.partneringinsuccess.com

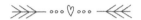

There is beauty in finding the silver lining, even through the darkness. It is there if you search for it.

TRACEY EHMAN

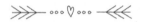

TAPPING INTO MIRACULOUS HEALING

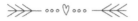

Winifred Adams

In my wildest dreams I could never have imagined that the "C" word would affect me. After all, I was the healer. I was the one helping others.

The day of my diagnosis was like a dream. I remember the living room of my apartment, with the light streaming through the multipaned windows and casting shadows on the wood floor. The noises outside were too loud as usual, with cars going by my Brentwood complex. I was on the phone with my gynecologist, listening to her tell me that I had dysplasia on my cervix and it required formal surgery, immediately.

I was wearing a long-sleeved white blouse and my favorite embroidered jeans with a peach-colored hummingbird stitched up the leg. At first, disbelief gave way to denial. There had to be a mistake. This wasn't my profile.

The office visit was imprinted in my memory. The nurse whom I had routinely seen each visit had a grim look on her face. My doctor then proceeded to take off the harmful cells on my cervix. This must be what a cat at the vet feels like, I thought. I hated this more than words could describe.

Humiliated and shamed, I was overwhelmed while feeling trapped in a situation I had no way out of. There was nothing left to do but resign myself to the diagnosis and the ultimate cause of this development in my life.

On my way home from the doctor's office, I placed a call to the man I referred to as my partner; only I knew better—he was my cheating partner. His denial and lack of care bolstered me in what would be my own journey ahead. Somehow, in that moment it all became crystal clear to me. I needed to drop the old and gear up for what I already knew to do for others—only this time it would be for me.

In my moment of clarity, driving alongside the picturesque Pacific Coast Highway, I realized the amount of work this would require, yet I was at ease. Something deep in my spirit told me that my journey was of value, both for myself and for many others yet to come. This was my golden thread of elixir that I would hold on to going forward.

Knowing full well how to heal and what to apply, I found myself weak. The kind of flippant disregard my partner had for my well-being made me feel as though I were swimming in mud. It was truly like being pinned by darkness. I reached out to another medical intuitive for insight, and she said, "I have never seen this before. It is like every cell in your body is spongy and not vital." Confirmed by blood work, I had fallen seriously ill, yet I still looked like a triathlete on the outside.

The day of my surgery was tough on me. My spiritual teacher's words echoed in my mind: "This is a gift, dear." The only solace I had were her additional words, and I clung to them: "There will be no more surgeries." The healer in me took her words to mean that I had a karmic payoff while Grace would work off the other amount. However, I'd been in the healing profession long enough to know what was ahead of me—I'd have to be sure the cancer didn't return and use herculean strength to overcome the negativity which had seeped into my system.

I had always known that having sex with someone is an exchange of energy, only now I learned that lesson as an indelible imprint upon my soul. After all, I believed in true love; only this wasn't loving. I simply could never again "exchange" energy if there wasn't love that cherished me in it. My system (as everyone's) would reflect the energy back to me, especially if it were not sincerely loving. To add insult to injury, my life had not been one of many careless flings like so many people experience. I was more careful and had always preferred one person at a time.

Coming out of surgery, I was in great pain. I will never forget the recovery room, where the only word I could muster was "pain." Another shot of something put me out again into numbness. A few hours later, I would walk out of the hospital, free of cancer, with all of my organs but missing part of my cervix. And something was profoundly clear to me: I felt new! I felt lighter, as if the surgeon hadn't just cut out cancer, but some rogue energy that was weighing me down. I felt wounded but rejuvenated.

A few weeks later, the next visit to my doctor was again met with a despairing look. The cancer had returned. In my mind, life seemed blurry. The surgeon was telling me that I would now lose my reproductive system, and likely would need to go on radiation or chemotherapy. I wanted to look behind me as if to say, "You can't be talking about me."

I looked at him and answered point blank, "Not a chance." And I got up and walked out in defiance.

That was when I decided to take to heart that, no matter how this came about, I was more powerful and would make the change in my own body. I knew how.

Blessing the doctors involved for their help, while acknowledging their limitation, I then took it upon myself to dig deep and heal myself. Day and night I engaged in the modality of "tapping." I used EFT as a means of undoing all the negative energy that had been in my body. Instead of my tendency to hold blame or resentment toward my former partner, I succumbed to forgiveness and release, instead. Once I felt clear of that energy, I meticulously went after the cells themselves, turning them around and interrupting their expression, which was not that of love. I was able to shift the expression altogether using tapping, meditation, and applying hands-on healing to myself—along with diet and supplements. By doing this, it turned the expression of my DNA receptors (epigenetic head) back into alignment, making my body that much stronger!

A few weeks went by, and my next doctor visit was slated to be a grim one, where the "next step" would be determined. Only, this time, they were in shock and had a hard time admitting that it had suddenly disappeared. There was no more cancer! Perplexed, they didn't know what to say. This time I smiled as I walked out.

There was no point sharing "how" this happened, because I knew it would fall on deaf ears. It was, in fact, my own private victory. A year later, HVP was officially out of my system, and ten years later, I am still cancer-free and HVP-free.

This was not "luck." This was *intentional change*, and it took a core shift on my part to undo what had been created. I believe God gave me the strength and faith to carry this healing forward. I was given the gift of healing since birth, and using it on myself would be my ultimate test of all tests, proving the power of the shift that can take place when we align with the light. It took extraordinary contemplation, self-honesty, and a hard look at my thoughts, behaviors, and most of all, my belief system.

What I did for my own healing was actually fairly scientific in its approach. Perhaps in a few more years, those who practice medicine will turn a corner and be able to better support and hold the belief that *change really can take place* using energy and natural healing modalities. I believe strongly that there is a place for allopathic medicine *and* the expertise of surgeons, along with diagnostic proof. But I also *know* there needs to be more belief in an unseen world of energy that holds the key to healing.

Since this time, I have helped countless numbers of people with my work. I have gone on to shrink tumors with distance and hands-on healing, "Making Lives Brighter™!" Many "miracles" have taken place in my work. I know that if a person really wants to heal and their karma aligns to that, they can heal more easily than our world would have us believe today. In my case, I found my golden elixir in personal value. I regained value both of myself and for those whom I'd yet to assist.

In my book *On the Road to Enlightenment*, I share my entire healing journey, showcasing the miracles and the power of the unseen world of energy. It is my wish that people learn to "tap" into their spirit and discover the "possibility" that lies within, because from that what we refer to as *miracles* are possible. I am living proof! I am certain that when we endeavor to tap into our deepest truth, we find the "Silver Lining" for ourselves, and this always leads to healing either the physical body, the spiritual body, or both.

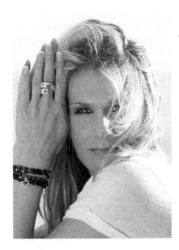

WINIFRED ADAMS *is a medical intuitive/master healer, radio show host, and professional wellness speaker for Making Life Brighter™. With the ability to see the origin of energetic imbalances, Winifred's rare but vast skill set shifts energy in Live-Time™, creating an environment for perfect and often complete healing. An expert in Extreme Healing™, Winifred, now shares her innate and unique gifts of intuition with audiences, creating an experience of Live-Time Healing™.*

www.makinglifebrighter.com

ONE LIFE

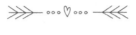

Jenna Auber

Surviving cancer gives me perspective daily. It has provided the opportunity to fight for everything I've ever held dear. It required that I dig deeper. It gave me permission to identify and make time for the people and activities I enjoy most—and to protect them like a lioness. In the face of fear and uncertainty, I allowed my diagnosis to empower me to upgrade my lifestyle, to let my light shine a little brighter, to dance in the rain, and to live every moment. In so many ways, life is sweeter than it's ever been.

It's been six years since I heard the words "you have cancer." I remember sitting in the doctor's office on my thirty-seventh birthday as though it were yesterday. As those words rang in my ears, I held my baby close, kissing his soft cheeks, cherishing his huge smile despite the gravity of the situation. I was young and healthy, feeling stronger than I had in years. There were no symptoms, no lumps. Had it not been for my aunt's diagnosis of ovarian cancer, and subsequently learning that I too carry the breast cancer (BRCA2) gene defect, my cancer would have gone undetected. As I sat there trying to absorb the impact of those gut-wrenching words, I immediately recognized that my aunt, genetic testing, and early screening had given me a fighting chance. I was grateful to have discovered the cancer when I did, and I shuddered to think what a few more years would have meant for my prognosis.

As I reflect on my cancer journey, it's as if it didn't even happen to me. Denial has been my close friend. I remember feeling determined to fight cancer from every angle and believing that I would absolutely make it to the other side of cancer treatment stronger than ever. But I became acutely aware that tomorrow is promised to no one. I desperately wanted to cherish every moment with my little ones, who were one and four at the time. Whenever possible, I focused my energy on positivity and gratitude. Day in and day out, I was in total awe of the way people rallied to support me and my family through the storm. Each act of kindness and generosity lifted my spirits and left me feeling loved, grateful, and full of renewed hope. But the truth is, it wasn't always pretty.

I remember some days feeling as though I'd lost a battle with a sledgehammer. The treatment left my body aching from head to toe making it difficult to even walk or enjoy my boys' sweet snuggles. Once an impressive multitasker, "chemo-brain" often left me feeling overwhelmed by every little thing. At times, for reasons I couldn't comprehend, my head would spin with rage, and my heart would break as my little ones took on the loving role of soothing me at bedtime.

With practice and a lot of self-compassion, I learned to sit with all the intense emotions that came with the diagnosis. There are still days when cancer leaves me feeling vulnerable and angry. It's robbed me of the ability to have more children.

It meant that I had to wean my baby from breastfeeding overnight. It took my hair, temporarily; my breasts, permanently. Embracing the silver lining and all the emotions that accompany a cancer diagnosis are not mutually exclusive. I've truly learned to feel, accept it all, and cherish the magic of every moment. I've learned to appreciate my inner strength, pick up the pieces, and keep moving forward.

I cherish and adore the little things more deliberately than ever: rubbing my sweet littles' backs each morning as we gear up to greet a new day and soaking in their precious snuggles and pillow talk each night. I breathe in gratitude and treasure my blessings. I pause to enjoy the warmth of the sun on my face, the wind blowing in my once-missing hair, the sound of the waves crashing on the beach or the birds singing, and that precious tiny hand in mine as we walk to school.

Remembering what it meant to me when faraway friends visited throughout treatment, I honor each year of survivorship with a trip to see people that mean the world to me. We sing, dance, climb mountains, laugh, and play. We celebrate all we have to be grateful for.

Whether I'm dripping sweat in a dark, music-filled spin room or enjoying the serenity of the open road, cycling is my "happy place," my refuge. Weeks after I completed treatment, I had the honor of "dancing" 111 miles on the bike in the pouring rain with Team Colleen, a nonprofit organization that helps cancer survivors accomplish a spectacular goal. The ride was cold, wet, and painful, but I smiled the entire way as I savored the air in my lungs, the power in my legs, and the support all around me. To this day, I love pushing my limits on the bike, annually choosing to climb 9,000 feet over 150 miles in a single day, telling the storm that is cancer, "Today, I shine!"

Five years after my cancer journey began, my brother called to share that he, too, was "joining the cancer club." It's a moment I will never forget. There was fear in his voice, but his words were brave as he tried to assure me that thanks to his broken hip, they'd caught it early. I worried his broken hip wasn't "luck," but evidence that the cancer had already made its way into his bones. I couldn't eat or sleep, fearing that his cancer journey might not look quite as mine had. He died two weeks later. In the blink of an eye, prostate cancer took my forty-five-year-old brother: a hardworking, playful, devoted single dad who was loved by all who had the honor of knowing his mischievous spirit and heart of gold.

In sharing our story, I'm realizing that my brother didn't need a brush with his own mortality to live his best life. Just today, I found something he'd written years prior to his diagnosis:

Take too many pictures, laugh too much, forgive freely, and love like you've never been hurt. Life comes with no guarantees, no timeouts, no second chances. You just have to live life to the fullest, tell someone what they mean to you and tell someone off, speak out, dance in the pouring rain, hold someone's hand, comfort a friend, fall asleep watching the sun come up, stay up late, be a flirt, and smile until your face hurts. Don't be afraid to take chances or fall in love and most of all, live in the moment. Dream what you want to dream, go where you want to go, be what you want to be because you have only one life and one chance to do all the things you want to do.

My brother did just that—and more. He was the silver lining in any storm, lifting the spirits of those around him with his quick wit and calm demeanor. He took the trip; always finding a way to make it home for the holidays or a Cape Cod summer. He was there in my time of need, rocking a bald head in solidarity, chasing our boys around the house until they fell to their knees in a fit of laughter. Being a father was his greatest joy in life. He took his son to Disney for his seventh birthday, a trip he arguably couldn't afford. It proved to be the last birthday he'd spend with his son.

My brother didn't wait for a diagnosis of cancer to recognize the beauty of life and what was important to him. He proclaimed that "life is a beautiful thing to cherish," and he made each day count.

I'm still working my way through the year of "firsts" after his death, oscillating between raw, painful grief and numb disbelief. I wish that, like me, we had caught his cancer early. Perhaps if we had known sooner, he would have had a fighting chance. I carry him with me in my heart wherever I go. I live to honor him and everything he represented. I recognize that had it not been for my aunt and genetic testing, my story could be the same as his.

It is my hope that in sharing our story, I can empower others with life-saving knowledge. I feel compelled to shout it from the mountaintops. In addition to breast and ovarian cancer, the BRCA gene defect includes an increased risk of prostate cancer. Emily Dickinson said, "If I can stop one heart from breaking, I shall not live in vain." I hope others can learn from our family's loss and take action to prevent their own heartache. If just one life can be saved as a result of genetic testing and early screening, my brother's death will not have been in vain. If just one person reads this and gets the upper hand on a cancer diagnosis, his light and the silver lining will shine as brightly as ever.

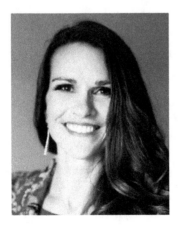

JENNA AUBER *is a passionate and dedicated labor and delivery nurse in Rhode Island, but being "Mom" is her most cherished role in life. She enjoys smiling until her face hurts, snuggling and playing catch with her little ones, cycling, dancing, chasing goals, and making each day count.*

HOW CANCER INFECTED MY FAMILY

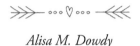

Alisa M. Dowdy

I was unaware that my grandmother had survived breast cancer before it ultimately took her life at the age of eighty-two. I came to understand that seven out of twelve members of her household were stricken by cancer in some form. The disease took the lives of five of her children (including my father). It also claimed the life of my brother, and it infected a few other close family members.

It's almost unbelievable how cancer can creep in without any noticeable indication until it's almost too late. Some people go on with their everyday lives until that one doctor visit that informs them of the grave news.

My father was a long-distance truck driver, traveling across the United States. He would call me at least twice a month or come by so he could show off his diesel truck to my neighbors. He enjoyed how people's faces would light up when he would roll up in his shiny big rig. Mainly, he wanted to assure me that he was living well.

I can't remember a time that I ever saw him sick. If he had a cold, it didn't last long, and if he was in pain, he never displayed his discomfort. He lived life looking and feeling healthy while he worked long, hard hours.

During his mother's funeral, I could see something in my dad's eyes. It was more than just grief from his loss. I could tell he wasn't quite himself. He seemed as if he had something to tell me, but he just kept insisting that everything was fine. He later told me that he was nursing a chest cold, but he was sure it wasn't anything serious. I think he knew there was something very seriously wrong with him, but he didn't want to face the truth. I eventually found out that he was self-medicating with over-the-counter cold medications in hopes that his "chest cold" would subside.

During this time, I had disturbing dreams of saying goodbye to him lying in a casket. I was so devastated I had to call my mother to tell her about them. She said she believed it was God's way of preparing me for what was to come. I tried to talk my dad into to seeing a doctor for a checkup. Whenever I called, he would promise me that he would make an appointment. Next, he would make appointments but purposely miss them. I believe he was afraid that he, too, would find out that he was going to die, just like his mother.

As a result, he didn't know he had a very serious condition that needed attention until it was too late. When he found out he had lung cancer, he had been hospitalized somewhere in North Carolina. The doctors told him to get back to family as fast as he could.

When he called me, I couldn't see him spending his last days anywhere other than with me. I cared for him the best I could. I remember him telling me that the breakfast I cooked for him one morning was the best he'd ever had. All I could do was smile and say, "I'm glad you liked it." I watched as he tried try to hold the water pitcher so he could pour himself a glass, but he ended up dropping the entire pitcher on the floor, which shocked us both.

At first I thought, He'll be fine. But as time went on, he became weaker and weaker. The man I considered to be the strongest man on earth was deteriorating right in front of me. Being only twenty-eight, I couldn't understand how this disease could infect and destroy my dad's body and then take him from me so quickly. I couldn't imagine my life without him. My mind couldn't comprehend life without his guidance and protection. My worst fears were realized on February 16, 1994. He passed ten weeks after coming to live with me. He was only forty-eight years old.

My brother was also forty-eight when he passed from pancreatic cancer. We were the same age for ten days. He was born in January, my mother conceived me in March, and I was born at the end of December. This made us feel like twins. We did everything together when we were young. We were in the same grade from first grade through high school. We even double-dated. We had a bond that only twins could comprehend, in spite of not having the best brother and sister relationship as adults. He went into the hospital on his birthday. He stayed there for nine days before the doctors told him he only had days to live. Cancer claimed his life thirteen days after his birthday in 2013.

After my father passed, his brother was like a father to my brother, sister, and me for twenty-years. I called him "Uncle

Pop." When he was diagnosed with lung cancer, he was given the option to have part of his lung removed. He had trouble deciding whether to go ahead with the surgery or not. He asked me what my father had done. My answer: "He died." So my uncle decided to have the surgery. He was in remission for a few years before the cancer returned and claimed his life at the age of sixty-seven in 2015. I felt as if I had just lost my father all over again.

The pain from all these losses has been overwhelming. How would I get through holidays, birthdays, or anything else that would remind me of them: a scent, a sound, a movie, a song, or the aroma of a Southern Style home-cooked meal that made up the precious moments we once shared over quiet family weekends and other special occasions.

How could I get past the grief? Some people burn candles around their loved one's pictures. Some like to tell their favorite stories that still make them laugh. Others cling to a favorite item that once belonged to their lost loved one. I found comfort in knowing that my grandmother, father, brother, and uncle were no longer suffering from the pain that cancer caused them. They have often visited me in my dreams with smiles on their faces to let me know that they are in a better place and at peace.

One thing is for sure, we never really get over the loss of a loved one. We grieve for however long it takes for our hearts to heal after such loss. We do the best we can to not let depression or sorrow overwhelm us. I learned that it is OK to move on and be happy; I can continue on with my life without guilt. I can choose to live my life differently than my family members did in order to prevent myself from enduring the same fate. I awaken each morning with the peace of mind that, although cancer infected my family, a piece of each of them will always be a part of my prevention. Getting past these losses is extremely difficult, but holding my loved ones in my heart has helped me heal.

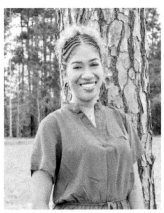

ALISA M. DOWDY *was born in New Jersey but raised in Oklahoma with two other siblings. She started writing at a young age. After becoming a mother of four her passion for writing was put on hold. In 2010, she was able to self-publish her first novel,* Before Dawn, *with anticipation of many more to follow. She enjoys writing, spending time with her family, and traveling. She now lives in Louisiana pursuing a career in motivational speaking.*

www.amdowdybooks.com

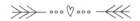

Loss makes artists of us all as we weave
new patterns in the fabric of our lives.

GRETA W. CROSBY

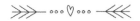

WINGS TO FLY

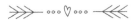

Erica Harris

The word *cancer* inherently denotes one dark cloud over-head; one full of worry, hurt, loss, hardship, and grief. It brings with it unimaginable indignities. Yet it's only in the face of such adversity that we come to see our own true colors for the very first time. And it's only after the stormiest of days that we have the chance of finding the very brightest of rainbows. My cancer journey was an Armageddon of storms, but it was also *that* journey that led me to shine brighter and bolder than I ever imagined possible.

In the early days of my cancer diagnosis, I constantly asked myself what I did wrong for cancer to have seeped in. But now I ask myself what I did right. I embarked on this path as a caterpillar. But through every bit of resolve, resilience, and fortitude, I emerged as a butterfly. With my newly gifted wings, I not only learned to take flight—I truly learned to soar.

I am now a well-versed, highly seasoned survivor—not only of an expected two-month terminal cancer prognosis, but also as the humbled and honored recipient of a bone marrow transplant and subsequently, a double lung transplant. All of which transpired over a ferocious three years in my mid-thirties. I was knocked down again and again and again, and yet there was a burning fire deep within to rise up, against the odds. Maya Angelou's powerful words, "Still, I rise" are now engrained within my very soul.

In my "previous life," I had always been passionate about health and wellness and had established a very successful career as a thriving sports chiropractor. I owned and operated my own multidisciplinary clinic. I loved inspiring others to attain their best health status, and I practiced what I preached. I hiked up mountains and soared down them on my skis. I was happily married and was an active young mama to two wee, precious boys. So I was absolutely aghast to learn that I was somehow very sick at the young age of thirty-five, while still nursing my youngest.

I sat stunned hearing the words of my shocking diagnosis of Acute Myeloid Leukemia (AML) after a routine lab test. In this instant, time literally seemed to pause. As I gazed out the window overlooking the bustling downtown city streets below, my attention was captured by an energetic woman walking along the sidewalk, sporting a bright yellow backpack and white sneakers. She walked with such spunk in her step, her dark hair bouncing as she greeted others cheerfully in passing. It was the same route I had walked many times before, with that very same spunk and that very same ear-to-ear smile. At that moment I was overwhelmed with the reality of just how lucky we all are to get to engage in those simple, everyday routines we so often take for granted.

As the stark reality of my catastrophic diagnosis set in, that vivacious woman provided powerful inspiration for all that was still to unfold on my journey. With every trying moment, I envisioned her spunk and her smile, and I fought to regain that same spirit in myself again.

Life as I knew it would never be the same. A bed was made available for me within hours at our province's largest hospital. With my head spinning, I was utterly clueless as to how to explain what we had just learned with my two tiny boys, just two and not yet five. I shared that we all have fighters to fight colds and bugs but that mama's fighters were not as strong as they needed to be. As we left for the hospital, my littlest angel passed me a treasure he had collected from the beach—a very special heart-shaped rock. It is still my lucky charm today. My big boy spontaneously shouted out loud and proud, with his huge, beaming smile, "Go, fighters, go!" That message of empowerment instantly became my mantra, one that has hurdled me through the most gruelling of moments and is still a resounding inspiration on my path today.

I spent the next two months as an inpatient undergoing a harsh chemotherapy regimen. My arms and legs were covered in bruises from spending days on end in a fetal position while retching endlessly. I endured multiple rounds of septic infections with dangerously high fevers. I was kept alive by 24/7 IV medications and constant transfusions made possible by the kindness of strangers. I lost all ten fingernails and all ten toenails, along with all my hair. The long nights brought terrifying nightmares and drenching night sweats.

I had an 80 percent chance of responding to the first round of treatment. However, my leukemic cells only soared, nearly doubling. "Salvage" chemotherapy was my only chance for remission, and only once in remission would I be eligible for a much-needed bone marrow transplant. My only brother proved not to be a match and a worldwide exhaustive search was hailed to find a suitable donor. After weeks of waiting for good news, a perfect match was finally established. I was filled with hope. I knew in my heart that I would not only survive but thrive.

However, not even twenty-four hours later, I received the crushing news that the salvage chemotherapy had not been successful. I was not in remission and thus no longer eligible for this bone marrow transplant. The gift of the life, extended just the day before, was now out of reach.

Instead I was awarded a terminal prognosis with two months to live. And yet, I held on to one thread of hope: this perfectly matched donor just waiting for me to do my part and rise up. I set forth on a mission to stay healthy enough to convince someone, somewhere in the world, to grant me this transplant without first being in remission. This became my fight of fights.

I pursued any and everything in the natural healthcare realm, from spiritual healing and meditation to green juicing and vitamin supplementation. We were enveloped with love and prayers from forces worldwide. I read self-help books, and one in particular had a pivotal impact. I was inspired by the words of Dr. Bernie Siegal, a medical doctor who encourages the practice of visualization in his book, *Love, Medicine, and Miracles*. I pictured myself walking across my graduation stage of health as he recommended. I envisioned wearing my cap and gown, receiving my diploma for having conquered cancer, and I instantly beamed with feelings of pride and joy.

After reflecting on that vision, I turned my gaze back toward the photos I was holding. I was in the process of making memory books for my two sons. I realized I was holding two photos of myself—one receiving my diploma from the University of British Columbia, and the other during my valedictorian address at my chiropractic school graduation. This served as a profound "aha" moment, shining a light on my survival. I knew this was a sign that I would one day walk across my own graduation stage of health.

Miraculously, I did get healthy and I even attained remission! Plans for me to undertake the anticipated transplant began immediately.

On the night I was readmitted for transplant, fireworks lit up the skyline of Vancouver over Stanley Park. I had no clue why fireworks were going off in mid-October, but it was another profound sign that I was in the right place at the right time. I later learned it had been the Leukemia and Lymphoma Society's annual event, "Light the Night" that lit my own night!

I grew stronger again. I was back to yoga, hiking, and teaching my young boys to ski. I biked, I rollerbladed, and I crossed finish lines, all while smiling ear to ear.

This burst of health, however, proved to be short-lived. Despite my physical strength improving daily, my cardiovascular strength seemed to be on a steady decline. I was literally running out of air. My new immune system was rejecting my own lungs. My weight dropped to 88 pounds, and I needed full-time oxygen.

And then, I received "THE" call that saved my life—exactly

three years to the day of receiving my terminal prognosis. My very worst day became my very best day, and my new lungs set me afloat.

On this journey, my husband was an incredible support, but the trials and tribulations all proved too great for my once-happy marriage to withstand. Yet, only after losing everything was I able to gain what I didn't even know I was missing. Cancer gave me my wings, but I was the one who had to grow them.

Despite the many undeniable hardships, I have been infinitely blessed by this turbulent cancer journey. I carry a new lightness in my heart and profuse gratitude for every moment. My heart has been set aglow, and I am now soaring to new heights. But the biggest gift of all is that I "get" to be mama to two of the most precious, resilient, and empathic little souls!

Live, Laugh, Love!

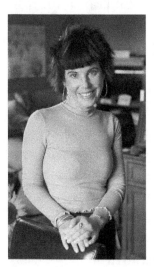

DR. ERICA HARRIS, *a well-versed, highly seasoned survivor, serves as an inspirational speaker and a patient advocate. She is a retired sports chiropractor and kinesiologist having previously owned, operated, and sold her own multidisciplinary clinic. She volunteers with the Canadian Leukemia and Lymphoma Society and the West Coast Kids Cancer Foundation. Erica is a proud supporter of Canadian Blood Services and on the board of directors for Zili Health.*

www.withhope.ca

THE 13 BLESSINGS FROM MY UNEXPECTED JOURNEY

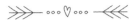

Kathryn F. Lininger

Hello, friend. We share something in common: the shock and awe of facing an unexpected journey, donning our battle armor for a fight we have not trained for. It is an adventure of self-pity, fear, finding a support network, and beginning a "new normal."

I am a two-time stage III cancer "thriver." I had a tumor removed through a craniotomy in my parietal brain lobe, and three years later it returned elsewhere, resulting in a right mastectomy and subsequent chemotherapy and radiation. Seven surgeries later I am telling my story.

My journey began in 2010 when I was forty-five years old. I repeatedly woke up at night short of breath. I visited a nurse practitioner who said my oxygen saturation levels were normal and sent me home. Eventually my dog woke my spouse when I was in the middle of a seizure, resulting in a 911 ambulance arriving at my doorstep. The emergency room informed me I had a growing tumor crowding my brain and causing pressure—the answer to my shortness of breath and seizures.

My insurance had contracted brain surgeons listed in their

network, but I located the top brain surgeon from UCSF. I sent him an email with my MRIs, and he agreed to perform my "awake" brain surgery to remove the tumor. I was prepared to start a "GoFundMe" account, but my insurance miraculously authorized him (blessing number 1)!

I took oral chemotherapy for ten months. The fear of surviving a brain tumor and coming out OK was terrifying. I did experience expressive aphasia and a yearlong lisp, but they both resolved after speech therapy. It took me about a year to recover and return to running my business out of my home office, carefully reviewing my work three times.

Three years later I was diagnosed with breast cancer and had an immediate mastectomy, followed by IV chemotherapy and radiation. This resulted in hair loss and the inevitable cachexia—a state of emaciation from the weak wasting of the body. The chemotherapy wiped out my entire body, getting rid of both the good and bad "soldiers"; the idea was that I would start from square one once the cancer cells were killed off. I worked from home in my bed.

During the chemotherapy I ordered two wigs. My thick, curly auburn hair fell out in chunks before they arrived. My dark blue crocheted hat soon became my best friend. One advantage of going bald was that I could pick out the hair I've always wanted: a bone-straight strawberry blonde asymmetrical bob! No more bad hair days! Going bald gave me the hair I've always dreamed of (blessing number 2)! Note to self: ALL hair disappears, including eyebrows and eyelashes, which are important since they protect and prevent particles in the air from going into one's eyes. One final hair note: my hair came back dark brown instead of auburn, still curly but baby fine; it's now the perfect texture of relaxed waves I had wanted my whole life without requiring a straight perm (blessing number 3)!

Shock was my first response after receiving the news that the biopsy of the brain tumor and breast biopsy were *not* benign. I immediately thought it was a death sentence. My physicians, neurologists, nutritionists, and oncologists were the bearers of bad news, offering blood transfusions, consultations, MRIs, and so on. Soon I went from one physician to *nineteen*, each with different specialties and suggestions for my course, including a geneticist.

There is a tendency to wallow in our sorrows when we realize our lives are at stake. I swam in the pity-party swimming pool for a short period. Since I had two teenagers, a business to run, and a spouse who found a new relationship during my second diagnosis, there was little time for this.

During my treatment I was delighted to have *unexpected angels* come my way: the postal carrier who came down my driveway every day to hand-deliver my mail, the UPS driver who picked pomegranates from my tree and put them on my picnic table, my old employee who baked me a polenta casserole, my friend who felt the "pull" of God telling her to stop by. Although I hid the fact that I had a recent mastectomy, she became a listening ear and is now one of my best friends. My brother and his wife stayed with me for seven months to help me during chemotherapy—a Godsend! Thank you, God, for these wonderful unexpected angels you sent me out of nowhere (blessings 4, 5, 6, 7, and 8)!

Eventually I realized that I was still getting out of bed each day, my feet were hitting the floor, I was walking and talking . . . I was still alive! I can work, exercise, and help people in some capacity. This makes me feel good. It's time to pull myself up by my bootstraps, and I'm not talking about Cinderella's glass slipper. I learned how to get out of my daily pity-party by thinking of someone I could help. I soon realized that there was no time to wallow because I was in a hurry to repair myself. Each time I felt sorry for myself, I would immediately find a speaker to listen to who would uplift me or find someone who needed help even more than I did. This got the attention off myself. I learned that as long as I'm breathing and functioning, I have work to do, my purpose to fulfill. I also wanted my children to know I could be strong, so they could focus on high school and college. My son and daughter took it upon themselves to support me through walks and runs for cancer research. My son wore a breast cancer pin on his backpack and pink on his football uniform during breast cancer month. My daughter became an RN through all of this (blessings 9 and 10)!

I learned to get busy doing something, no matter how small. I need to "keep on keepin' on." It's time to put on my track shoes, dig my cleats in, get some traction, and hit the ground running toward ongoing recovery. After all, I am still alive! It's time to put on the brakes, stop, and make a u-turn in order to improve my previous lifestyle.

Now I have a new normal. I am constantly in a state of

renewing my body to combat it rather than have it combat me. My new wonderful spouse is 100 percent on board, and he is my top life coach along with my daughter who is a progressive care nurse (blessings 11 and 12)! For the past nine years I have been studying health, including natural herbs and essential oils.

If you are a coach like me, pick your team members and have them surround you in your personal space. Have them coach you: What are you eating and drinking? Are you exercising? Are your pantry and refrigerator cleaned out? Have you gotten rid of all the sugar in your house, or are the wrong foods still tempting you? Eventually you will weed out what causes inflammation or a leaky gut. Invite them to closely inspect your life, making sure you are putting the right things in your body so you can be healed. They are your accountability partners. Remember, they are there to keep you on the right course. These coaches will become healthy along the way too, so you will benefit from each other. Remember, we become like who we surround ourselves with, and we wear off on each other. The whole household can turn around if one person takes the helm at the food court!

Exercise can do wonders for your brain power. While enjoying nature, you can listen to a speaker or some uplifting music. You can talk to God and admire His beautiful creation. During one of my neighborhood "walks," I was complaining to God about how I wouldn't have enough money to make the next payroll. I looked down and saw a small "painted rock" in the ditch among other larger rocks. It had been painted by an extremely skilled artist and featured a beautiful angel with red hair, like mine used to be. She had a yellow halo, white wings, a blue flowing gown, and small beads around her neck. When I picked up the rock, I thanked God for giving me a gift I could see and hold (blessing number 13)!

I'm still alive! I will keep moving forward, reaching out to others and helping them, keeping it simple, pacing myself, considering decisions carefully, and bouncing them of my core people. And more blessings are sure to follow!

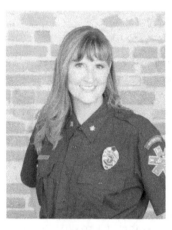

KATHRYN F. LININGER *served as the founder and commander in chief of TLC Emergency Medical Services from 1999 to 2019. She holds three college degrees and is certified in Occupational Therapy and Emergency Medical Dispatch. She serves as a team lead for the GO-TO-OT Advocacy Initiative for the Occupational Therapy Association of California and works in skilled nursing and home health settings. Kathryn offers training and education, public speaking, community outreach, and advocacy for seniors and access and functional needs populations.*

www.pointmenow.com

I AM BRAVE AND I AM STRONG

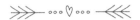

Susie McQueen

In the summer of 2012, my kids and I were staying with my parents at their cottage. I woke up one morning and realized that my vision was gone. My eyes were open, but all I could see was darkness. Over the course of a few minutes, I could see light as my vision slowly returned. It felt as if I was looking through a small tunnel that gradually expanded.

My fitness and health has always been an important part of my life. I probably should have remained quiet, but I continued to move forward with my daily Shaun T Insanity Workout by video. Following my workout, my head began to pound. The pain was so intense that it knocked me to my knees, as tears ran down my face. My mom has a history of migraines, so I did not think much of it. Later on, I found out that this excruciating headache was the result of the left side of my brain swelling and putting pressure on the right side of my brain.

In order to try to get some pain relief, I made a massage appointment for the next day. I borrowed my dad's truck and drove myself into town. At my destination, I stepped out of the truck and fell straight on the ground. I lost all control of my legs, and I was unable to form any words. As I lay frightened on the ground, I looked for someone, anyone, to help me. There was not a soul in sight. I am not sure how long I was unable to move, but when I regained control of my legs, I got up and continued on to my appointment.

The next day I decided to visit my eye doctor, as my vision continued to bother me. After examining my eyes, the doctor sent me to the ophthalmologist on call at the local hospital. He examined my eyes and took photos of the optic nerves at the back of both eyes. Normally optic nerves look like tiny pinpoints, but mine looked like giant starbursts. The doctor said that the optic nerves were enlarged because there was too much pressure on them. When I asked him if I might have a brain tumor, he quickly replied that he was 99.9 percent sure that I did not. After all, I was a very fit, healthy young woman. He said he would request an MRI to see what was causing the pressure.

As soon as we arrived back at the cottage, my mom, who was worried about waiting for an MRI, phoned a very close friend who happened to be the head of oncology at the local hospital. Although he was on vacation, he arranged to see me the next morning. I had an MRI at noon, and he saw me for a follow-up appointment that afternoon. He was so concerned that he insisted that I leave my mom's car in the parking lot while he drove me to our cottage himself. He also contacted my dad and instructed him to close his office immediately as he wanted us to travel to London that night.

He arranged for me to be admitted to the University Hospital in London upon arrival. No one remembers hearing that I had a brain tumor, although he insists that he told us— perhaps we were incapable of absorbing that information at the time.

It was a wild and crazy scene while we packed up all of the gear for my 4 month old son and 2 year old daughter. We literally hurled everything into my Dad's truck. Dad and I sat in the front seats, while Mom was squeezed between 2 giant car seats in the back. Mom's big Black Lab was stretched out on the floor of the back seat. We left the cottage at 8:00 pm and drove through the night arriving in London at 5:00 am.

Mom recalls that I was amazed at the two giant moons in the sky that night. I didn't realize that I was seeing double! She was also amazed that I was so wakeful and chatty, keeping my Dad alert as we journeyed on. No one understood that the pills I was taking every four hours were massive doses of Decadron, a powerful steroid that was busy reducing the swelling in my brain. It is known for causing insomnia!

When we arrived in London, my mom took the kids and the dog back to the house, while my dad came with me to the hospital.

As I sat in the hospital, awaiting a bed, I remember hoping that there would not be a bed for me. I wanted so badly to retreat to my cosy home where I could feel safe again. Once I was settled in my uncomfortable hospital bed, the doctors seemed to come from everywhere. I felt very overwhelmed as two different groups of doctors and their students came to talk to me. The frustration set in, as I had to answer the same questions multiple times. Finally, a doctor came in with a student. It was time to get my diagnosis. He asked if I wanted anyone to be with me when I received the news. I just wanted to get it over with. I tried to be strong; I took a deep breath and told him that I was ready for my diagnosis. My heart dropped as he told me that I had a brain tumor.

The first question that came to my mind was "Am I going to die?" I fought to hold back tears as I tuned out the rest of what the doctor was saying. After he finished talking, I asked if I could go home, but he told me that the tumor could cause me to have seizures during the night and staying in the hospital would be the safest choice for me. I curled up in a ball and cried like I had never cried before.

As soon as my husband, James, heard that I was in the London Hospital, he came right away. I was unable to explain what was happening as he held me in his arms. The hospital staff brought in an extra cot so that he could remain at my side.

Following my diagnosis, I underwent a craniotomy (brain surgery) in hopes of removing the tumor. After I returned from surgery, the doctors gave news that no one wants to hear. The tumor that sat in my brain was still there; the cancerous cells were closely intertwined with my healthy brain cells, making it impossible for successful removal. I was given two options moving forward: chemotherapy or radiation. I was determined to fight so I want my treatment to be aggressive. I decided to move forward with both chemotherapy and radiation, hoping to destroy the cancer that resided in my brain, unwelcomed. I also began to practice a Kundalini Yoga Mantra, designed to aid healing.

My traditional treatment began with radiation. The treatment itself did not take that long, but the aftermath was uncomfortable. I had what appeared to be a bad sunburn on my upper chest and the back of my neck. I also had the misfortune of developing what is known as "moon" face, which is the swelling of the face caused by ongoing doses of Decadron. I did what I could to hide it such as by wearing hats daily; however, it was still obvious to most people. In addition, my hair began to fall out. I remember clumps of hair falling out in the shower. As my hair continued to fall out, I decided that it was time to shave my head. My mom was visiting, so I asked her if she could shave my head for me. As I watched her take the shaver to my head, tears ran down my face and my hair fell to the ground. It was hard, but I knew that my hair would grow back—besides, pixie cuts were in!

Chemotherapy was much different. I expected to sit in a room with other people, fighting their fight, and go through the process of getting chemotherapy through IV. However, I was able to take pills at home. It made me so happy to not have to go to the hospital each day for my treatment.

My visits to the hospital for my MRIs have been stretched out from three months to six months to nine months. My last MRI was about eight or nine months ago now. At this point in my life, I am still unable to drive or return to work because of the potential for seizures. I do feel healthier and stronger than I have in the past. My family and friends have supported me throughout this process, and their continued support has been amazing as I continue to fight this diagnosis. I'd like to end with a statement that a friend wrote:

Each and every day, be Strong, be Positive,
be Supportive and, above all, Never, Ever, Ever quit
or give up hope. Never!

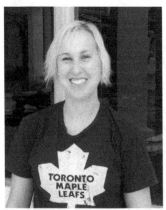

SUSIE MCQUEEN *grew up in Sault Ste. Marie, Ontario, and studied kinesiology at the University of McMaster. She loves the outdoors and enjoys spending time at her parents' cottage in Northern Ontario. She also has been a world traveler, snowboarder, and skier. She spent time in Costa Rica studying to be a yoga instructor, before becoming an elementary school teacher. She lives in London, Ontario, with the love of her life, James, and her two children, Lily and Eddie.*

HEALING WITH LOVE

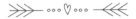

Lisa Manyon

"Do you think you have cancer?" This question stunned me. I was almost speechless that a healthcare practitioner would ask me this. There's a little thing like never going to medical school that precluded me from having the answer to this question. After all, I was there to get a professional opinion.

I knew something big was going on, but I didn't know what. My healthcare practitioner at the time insisted that what I was experiencing was an abscessed tooth. I *knew* that wasn't what it was, but I never in a million years imagined it was cancer. My airway was tightening, I was having trouble breathing and swallowing, and I could *feel* something growing in my throat.

This was April 2017. It would be weeks until I could get into the ENT (Ear Nose Throat) specialist. Weeks of wondering, *What if I do have cancer?* Thankfully, the divinely guided message I received was "You're going to heal this with love." I held on to faith with the occasional thought of *Am I being delusional? What if I die tomorrow?*

The truth is I was OK with either outcome. When I assessed my life, my life was rich. A quick inventory revealed that the only things I still wanted to accomplish were 1) publish my book(s); 2) go to Italy; and 3) visit the rain forest. Of course, I thought of my parents. I also thought of meeting my soul partner. But all in all, I was good with my life, and I still am. In fact, it's become even richer.

As I sat in inquiry, I said a prayer to thank God for my life, acknowledged that this was way bigger than me, and expressed my gratitude for everything I'd already experienced throughout this lifetime. I added "I'm OK with the outcome either way, but I'm really not ready to check out, and I think you have more work for me to do in this world." I settled into absolute faith that all would be exactly as it should be, and I followed divine guidance throughout the entire process.

In the United States, one in two women and one in three men will be diagnosed with some type of cancer in their lifetime. A recent study in the UK indicates that it's more like one in every two people. Cancer is not discriminating. There are more than one hundred types of cancer, and as you're reading this, that means either you or I have been diagnosed or will be diagnosed (statistically speaking). In this case it was me. On May 16, 2017, I heard the words, "You have cancer."... or it might have been "It is cancer."... either way, these three words are not words I'd wish upon anyone. Nonetheless, I did not let this define me, nor did I accept it as "mine", and I was determined to heal with love.

Instead, I embraced self-care and that became my number-one priority. It should be yours too.

Lisa Manyon

Healing with Love Transforms Everything

Taking control of my health and choosing ME has been an amazing journey and a true testament of faith. I encourage *you* to choose YOU so you can take control of your health and hopefully avoid any serious healthcare wake-up calls.

I underwent two major surgeries on August 10, 2017. I kept it quiet. I relied upon my sacred sphere of influence to be my support system, and I focused on embracing wellness. What I know for sure is that I am delighted to be a thriver. I prefer the term *thriver* over *survivor* because that's what I am. I turned my health around to thrive without chemo or radiation.

The cancer is now gone, and I am on a continuous healing journey. I've released forty pounds, eliminated all processed food, changed my entire life for the better, and continue to focus on healing with love.

I think Mother Teresa said it best when she said, "I will never attend an antiwar rally; if you have a peace rally, invite me." She had it dialed in. When we wage war on anything or rally against anything, or declare a battle to fight against something, we create more momentum for the very thing we are against. Words have energy, and my focus is healing with love.

I understand this may seem counterintuitive to most (welcome to my world), but it is pure truth. It's what I've been teaching in the context of my work, it's what Mother Teresa so eloquently shared with a simple quote, and it's what the world needs to course correct—*it is pure love.*

When we want to change something, we must engage in full-on LOVE, not wage war.

We must flip the script and focus only on the positive outcome.

We must take positive, proactive action instead of inciting riled-up reaction.

This is not a new concept. I cannot take full credit for it; I can only live it and invite you to do the same.

This doesn't mean we won't be challenged. This doesn't mean we won't get ticked off at circumstances. This doesn't mean that we won't feel despair based on world affairs.

We are human. We will *feel*. We will *live,* and hopefully we will *love*.

I believe we can heal anything with love. And to do that we must start somewhere.

With ourselves. With our families. With our friends. With our communities. With our world.

♥ Love yourself—treat yourself well; be kind.

♥ Love your family—which often means forgiveness and understanding.

♥ Love your friends—reach out and let them know how much they mean to you.

♥ Love your community—get involved; small acts have big impact.

♥ Love your world—take care of this precious resource we have been given.

And, yes, I know, life will rock you to the core. It may make you want to wage war, but remember: the only thing that ever really heals is love.

When we combine love with knowledge and action, we have the power to facilitate great change in the world.

My Top Lessons from Healing Cancer with L♥VE

1) Focus on *life*. When you push against anything, it creates more of what you don't want. It's important to focus on healing, not fighting, battling, or conquering. The language we use creates our reality.

2) You are 100 percent responsible for taking control of your health. Learn about nutrition, healthy eating, and how to fuel your body the right way.

3) Question everything. Get a second opinion (or more). Push for what you need. Don't take no for an answer.

4) Healthcare practitioners don't know everything. I was initially misdiagnosed. Had I listened, I wouldn't be writing this today. #truth

5) Doctors are valuable resources. They do stay in their lane, though. So focus on what you know will improve your health beyond what the doctors tell you (research nutrition and real food). It took surgery and a complete dietary reset to heal with L♥VE.

6) People don't know how to deal with cancer. So when people do show up, it means a lot. More than you will ever know. When people don't show up, it hurts. More than *you* will ever know.

7) Cancer is becoming "normal." Let that sink in. There is nothing normal about this. That means it's up to you and me to boost our immune systems, eliminate toxins in our homes, reduce stress, eat more fruits and vegetables (preferably organic), eliminate processed poisonous foods, take the time to educate ourselves about what it takes to live a healthy life, and incorporate what we learn.

The truth is, we are not promised tomorrow.

When people showed up, it meant the world to me. For those who would have liked to show up but didn't know, I'm sorry. I had to keep this within the sacred sphere of influence, and when you're facing something like this, it's hard to reach out (especially when you do and . . . crickets).

Many have asked me to share what I did to turn my health around. It's important to know that every cancer is different, every person is different, and that means that what I did worked for *me*. It's not a guarantee for anyone else. We all must take our health into our own hands and make ourselves—and of course, our families—the priority.

For now, I'm simply grateful. Grateful for every breath. Grateful for those who bring peace and positivity into my life.

Grateful for my family, my friends, my health, my fabulous clients, and life.

I invite you to sprinkle a little "spiritual sugar" on your life by redefining your relationships with Self, Health, and Wealth. It all starts with you.

Every minute and every second is precious. Where are you starting with LOVE today?

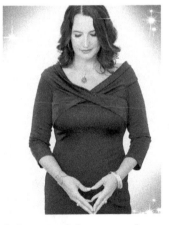

LISA MANYON *is the business marketing architect and president of Write On Creative®. She pioneered the three-step Challenge. Solution. Invitation™ framework to create marketing messages with integrity by focusing on PASSION points. Her strategies are known to create million-dollar results. She is a cancer thriver who believes in healing with L♥VE. She shares her personal story, journal prompts, and inspiration to help you redefine your relationship with self, health, and wealth via Spiritual Sugar™.*

www.SpiritualSugar.com

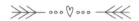

You are more powerful than you know;
you are beautiful just as you are.

MELISSA ETHERIDGE

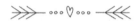

LIFE IS BEAUTIFUL

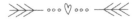

Nimira Mohamed

She sat in tranquility, her fingers gently moving the beads of her pearl prayer tasbi, one at a time, while she quietly chanted her prayers. Peace was reflected in the gentle outline of her face. Looking at her, one would never guess that she was in pain or discomfort. She was grace personified. Her name was Roshan, which means "shining light" in Sanskrit. She really was a shining light to everyone she met, always inspiring others with her optimistic attitude and beautiful smile. Her friends and contemporaries nicknamed her "Sukari," which means "sweet" in Kiswahili, and this, too, was reflective of her endearing personality.

After a routine mammogram, my mother, Roshan, was diagnosed with fourth-stage metastatic breast cancer in 1989. She was very particular about her health and had been going regularly for her mammograms. At first, she thought the doctor had mixed her results with someone else's—she had no symptoms, and she had received an "all clear" on her last mammogram. But the diagnosis was all too real. She was shocked, scared, and had a feeling of doom and disbelief. The cancer was terminal, she was informed, and her chances of survival were slim. There was no real cure. The diagnosis hit her like a storm, stirring up emotions and feelings that threatened to overwhelm her, but when the dust settled and she calmed down, she was determined, like a warrior, to put up a brave fight just as she had done at every stage of her life.

My mother had lost her parents at a very young age and became a mother to her two younger sisters. She was widowed at age thirty-five with six young children, and she became a refugee when President Idi Amin expelled all Asians from Uganda, forcing her to leave the country of her birth, a country she truly loved. She had to rebuild her life and those of her children in a completely new country. Life had dealt her many challenges, but she was not about to give up. Her unwavering faith in God, and her trust that He was with her every step of the way, kept her calm and resolute.

As recommended by her doctors, she aggressively pursued treatment with several bouts of radiation and regular chemotherapy in the hope that she could beat the cancer. Nobody gave up on her—not her doctors, not the cancer clinic, the hospital staff, and definitely not her family. Progress was always expected, no end date was stamped on her, and she never quit.

As Elisabeth Kubler-Ross said, "People are like stained-glass windows. They sparkle and shine when the sun is out, but when the darkness sets in, their true beauty is revealed only if there is a light from within." Even though the drugs administered through the chemotherapy made her feel nauseated and light-headed, she was always compassionate toward the people around her, always making them feel comfortable with her cheerful demeanor.

The one time she broke down was when tufts of her hair came off in her hands while she was showering, leaving her with bald patches on her head. Tears streaming down her face, she sobbed uncontrollably in shock as she came out of the bathroom. I hugged her, lost for words, murmuring soft words of comfort until she calmed down. After that time, she was back to her sanguine and calm self. I never heard her complain about her fate, the discomfort, or the pain. She was aware that my siblings and I were very concerned about her health, and she did not want to exacerbate that concern by complaining. On the contrary, she would bolster us and make our spirits rise out of despondency until we were smiling—dissipating for the moment the fear of losing her.

The treatments drained and exhausted her. She would barely recover from one chemo when it was time for another. Her journey was a marathon that took every ounce of her energy, not a sprint. Some days were good, and on others she was completely fatigued, spending a lot of hours sleeping to recover her strength. Despite the obstacles and adversity, she lived life to the fullest, focusing on making each lucid moment count—even traveling back to Africa to visit her place of birth.

Like all of us, my mother thought that death was something that would happen in the distant nebulous future, far away. After the diagnosis of MBC, it took center stage. Suddenly her life came into bright focus; every moment of each day was precious, not to be taken for granted. She swept away the cobwebs of unimportant things, making her world magical. Life was beautiful to her, and she looked at things we all take for granted as a blessing: the gentle wind on her face, the scent of the cherry blossoms, the snowflakes painting the landscape, her family's smiles. She even created a photo album for each of her grandchildren to remind them of how much she loved each one of them.

My mother passed away peacefully on Easter 1992. She was an inspiration to all of us. Through my life, as I face adversities, I look for the silver linings, as she did. Life is not about how long we live, but about focusing on our blessings and not taking any moment for granted. Her cancer made our lives more beautiful because we spent each moment we could together and made every day count. When time is short, the wind brushes away the unimportant things, leaving the world beautiful and bright. It is in the small things, those little moments of beauty that are so easy to overlook in the hustle and bustle of our busy lives, that we find peace and true happiness.

I just want to tell anyone who is going through cancer or knows someone who is going through it to stay positive! Every day single day that God gives us is a blessing. He doesn't put us through anything we can't handle. Every challenge makes us stronger. Live . . . love . . . hope . . . laugh . . . fight . . . pray. Enjoy every precious moment. Surround yourself with family and friends and make every moment count. Modern science now has many innovative cancer treatments, and new ones continue to be discovered all the time. Do your research, seek out the best treatment, and remain strong. But also don't forget to live and appreciate all that life has to offer. Life is about enjoying the journey, not just about reaching the destination. And there is always a light at the end of the tunnel—a silver lining in every cloud.

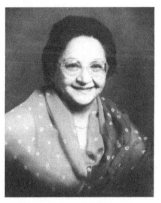

Roshan, Nimira's Mum

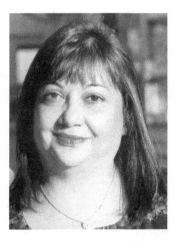

NIMIRA MOHAMED *is a beauty specialist, educator, and a licensed clinical spa esthetician. Nimira is passionate about making her clients feel beautiful inside and out. Nimira believes everybody deserves to feel beautiful at all times. She currently owns and operates Spa Willoughby in Langley, British Columbia, and she has also conducts skincare seminars in Las Vegas, Toronto, and Vancouver. Nimira is married and has a ten-year-old son, Aryz.*

www.spawilloughby.com

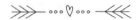

Keep your face to the sunshine and
you cannot see a shadow.

HELEN KELLER

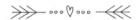

A FULL AND HAPPY LIFE

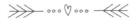

Lynn Pasquali

*If you had asked me twenty-five years ago when I first received my
cancer diagnosis whether I thought there was a silver lining,
I would have called you crazy.*

I wasn't sure I wanted to talk about my cancer because I
thought I might be tempting fate if I wrote it down, but
here is my story. I was in my forties, and my first daughter
had just gotten married earlier that year. My husband and I
had lots of plans of what we were going to do in the future,
including lots of traveling. Then one day, when I was doing
a self-exam, I discovered a small lump in my breast.

I made an appointment with my doctor, and he told me he
wasn't too worried about it, but that I should keep an eye on
it and record any changes. I think he just didn't want to scare
me, but I felt I couldn't leave anything to chance, and so, even
though I really liked my doctor, I asked for a second opinion
and a referral to a breast specialist. As I made the appointment,
I felt a sense of overshadowing doom, and I dreaded actually
going to the appointment. I didn't want to hear what I already
feared to be the case: that I had cancer. Unfortunately, I was
correct, and when the diagnosis was confirmed, my insides

57

turned to mush. I was scared and angry. I didn't know I could feel such conflicting emotions at the same time.

The specialist I saw was also a surgeon, and I had the operation within a week. Looking back now, it was a silver lining that there was so little time for me to think about it and instead just keep moving forward so the treatment could begin. The worst part about the operation was getting the drain removed a week or so later because the skin had grown around the tube. The oncologist advised me to have chemo and radiation to ensure that all the cancer cells were obliterated, even though there was no sign of cancer in the lymph nodes that were removed. I was cancer-free, but my journey wasn't over.

I had a total of four chemo treatments over a sixteen-week period. When I went for my first chemo session, I was surprised to see that I wasn't the youngest woman there. I saw women in their thirties also receiving chemo, and at that time, you didn't hear about younger women getting breast cancer. It was considered more the norm that women in their sixties or seventies were more at risk.

Receiving chemo by intravenous was a surreal experience. The room contained five or six "recliners" for the patients to sit in. The technician inserted the intravenous needle and I sat there for thirty minutes while the chemo entered my system. The first day after the treatment I was very sick, but it gradually subsided by the second or third day. During the two weeks in between treatments, I basically felt normal. As treatment went on, I experienced other side effects, such as canker sores, but they subsided when treatments ended. One thing that didn't subside or return to normal right away, however, was losing my hair.

After I recovered from the chemo, I had ten radiation sessions. Unlike the chemo, the radiation didn't take long; the actual session took about ten minutes. The people at the cancer clinic were a wonderful, caring group, and when I had my last treatment, they said they had enjoyed my company but hoped they wouldn't see me again. And you know what—they didn't! When I began losing my hair, I found a nice wig to wear until my own hair started growing back. That was a bit of a silver lining, too, because the wig I bought was a longer style than I normally wore, and it actually suited me better, so I have never had really short hair again. These days there are wig donations and much more support while you are going through this. The only thing they had when I had cancer were scarfs or ugly synthetic wigs that really didn't do much for anyone, but I persevered until I could find something that was OK. If I wasn't wearing my wig, I wore a baseball cap. My natural hair color was dirty blonde, but when it finally grew back in, it was black with very tight curls. Over time, though, the roots lightened up, and about a year later everything was back to almost normal.

One of the best feelings was being able to drive again because it was so liberating. I didn't have to depend on someone else anymore to get around. That might seem like a small thing, but for me it was huge. It meant I was returning to normal, and I could try and put the bad stuff behind me. I had lots of support from my family. My husband was amazing, and I probably couldn't have gotten through it without his support. While our travel plans were delayed a bit, some of my best holidays were after cancer—New Orleans Mardi Gras, New York, Hawaii, Italy, and numerous others.

I have seen both my daughters married, and I have four beautiful grandchildren, three of whom have graduated from high school, so that is definitely a silver lining. I wish I could say I changed my life, but as far as I was concerned, I was already living a great life before cancer struck. Once I was healed, I was grateful to have my normal life back, except for the annual checkups which were a reminder each year. I'm still my old goofy self, and that will never change. I get annoyed sometimes trying to fit a bathing suit as the lumpectomy resulted in an indent in an inopportune place, but other than that everything else is normal. I still have lots of curl in my hair, so it makes my fine hair a lot easier to manage.

The scariest thing about cancer is the diagnosis and then the prognosis, but after that it's time to get down to business and take care of it the best you can. I was one of the lucky ones, and if you are diagnosed now, you have an even better chance of surviving and having a full and happy life.

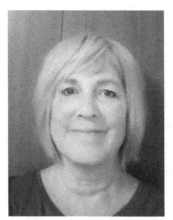

LYNN PASQUALI *is a loving wife, mother, and grandmother with an enviable enthusiasm for life. She was compelled to contribute to this book because she not only has a cancer-thriver story to share, but she also wanted to support her daughter, Tracey Ehman, and inspire others impacted by cancer.*

THE GREATEST BLESSING

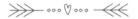

Deborah Reynolds

L ife has some interesting twists and turns. Life has highs, lows, exciting moments, tragic moments, laughter, sadness, calm, chaos, peace, and tranquility. Life is unpredictable. In September 2011 I was diagnosed with Chronic Lymphocytic Leukemia (CLL). I went for my annual physical and had my routine blood tests. When I viewed my blood reports online, I noticed that the white blood cell count and the lymphocytes were slightly above the normal range. I was curious and searched online for more information about lymphocytes. There were multiple causes listed which would result in a high reading and, being diligent, I followed up the next morning with a call to the doctor's office and made an appointment.

After reviewing my blood levels over the past few years, the doctor wasn't too concerned, so I shared with him what I read online. What caught my attention was that "CLL could be but was not necessarily related to Multiple Myeloma"— my father's diagnosis. I told the doctor, "There must be a test I can take to confirm whether I have cancer or not." He said, "Yes, it's a flow cytometry." *Push, Deb! Use your voice and stand up for yourself.* I realized in that moment how often I pushed for others; I was an advocate for the weak and vulnerable, but I wouldn't always push or fight for myself. I insisted on scheduling this test because it's important not to bury our head in the sand when it comes to our own well-being. We must take responsibility for our own health and life.

The results came back positive for CLL. The doctor explained that CLL was one of the slowest growing cancers. "The prognosis is fifteen to thirty years," he said. *Seriously? I'm planning to live another forty-plus years!* My next thought was, *How do I use this to help others?* I was being true to my giving spirit.

The diagnosis has certainly given me food for thought and forced me to revisit my life: what I was doing, how I was thinking, where I was putting my focus and energy. I believe perspective and attitude is everything. Being a realist, I knew I had to help myself first, before helping others.

I view this diagnosis as my greatest blessing! Not the cancer—the diagnosis! It woke me up and gave me the gift of deepening my spiritual walk and focus. My husband, Ken, asked me if I was afraid. I said, "No, I'm fascinated. Fascinated that my body would do this, and I want to know why." Then I went into research mode instead of burying my head in the sand.

My personal library, already massive, grew even more. I added more books on health and nutrition. I read Anita Moorjani's book, *Dying to Be Me*. I devoured it in a day, amazed by the similarities of our painful path. And like Anita, I found that every book I consumed on nutrition contradicted with every other health book. It felt like I was going in circles and not making any progress. I consulted with Pamela McDonald, creator of the APOE Gene Diet. She was Dr. Wayne Dyer's nutritionist. He also had CLL and had the same gene factor as mine. My conclusion, after all the reading, was a determination and commitment to clean up my life, my body, and my business. When I analyzed all the research, I focused on "inflammation." My body was sensitive, and I had been experiencing swelling around my eyes and face and stiffness in my hands. Foods and certain environmental products such as sprays irritated my body and lungs. And certain aspects of my life also were irritating me.

My life and my business have always been about helping others and adding value. My goal in business has always been to exceed people's expectations, and my clients constantly affirm my high value. My intention in life has been to leave each relationship better than what it was after engaging with people. Yet some people in my personal life had expectations of me that I could never meet, and in my attempt to please them, I became exhausted, frustrated, angry, and resentful. I was used and abused. I had to learn that you can't please people—and I had to get clear about who I am and how I want to show up in the world.

At my core I am loving, generous, kind, and compassionate, but if I choose to repress those beautiful parts of me and pull back because someone isn't treating me well, then I'm not being authentic. Loving from a distance became my motto—learning to forgive and release, sending them loving prayers and blessings, and standing in gratitude for all that life has given me was a much healthier mindset. I did not want to be angry and resentful. Peace was my goal.

So many of us desperately need to move inward and

experience more quiet time and self-reflection. We are seeking peace of mind and a renewed energy to love ourselves and our life. We can be too consumed with what is going on outside ourselves, worried about what others are thinking about us and what we are doing. The greatest joys in life come from doing the inner work. It is important to speak the truth, be authentically loving, keep your inner peace, and always be thankful. Peace of mind and a gentle up turning of the corners of your mouth come from going inward.

Being in control of your life is important, and making decisions from a calm, well-informed position is critical. But sometimes things are simply out of our control, and that is where the right attitude and perspective become necessary to attain that deep, quiet inner peace.

Then there is the aspect of "letting go and letting God take over." I began rethinking my life purpose. I equate this to a massive jigsaw puzzle, complete, but with the diagnosis, suddenly tossed into the air. Now I had to start all over again to define my life purpose and life plans. With time and deep reflection, everything became much clearer. Secretly, I was grateful for the time to reflect.

It was time for me to do a life review and get clear about my life, expectations, the contributions I wanted to make, how I wanted to spend my time, and with whom. Living with clarity was about loving acceptance of myself, being at peace with what I had endured in my lifetime, and feeling grateful for the woman I had become. It was about being, not striving. I realized I had enormous gifts to share and wanted to contribute.

My life has changed. I make sure there is less stress and plenty of rest and sleep. I have been focusing on the things I love to do, such as reading, playing the piano, and painting. I needed to clean up my body, lose weight, and hopefully eliminate inflammation. I removed my artificial nails, I stopped coloring my hair, and I found natural products for my body and natural household cleaners for my home.

My diet became more refined and healthier, and I now prefer home-cooked meals. I eliminated most sugars; I eat predominantly organic foods, organic free-range chicken, wild salmon, and occasionally grass-fed meat. I've added selective supplements and parasite cleansing, and I focus on removing heavy metals from my body. Meditation and prayer become part of my daily routine. I immersed myself more deeply in spiritual growth. I enrolled in a Yoga Teacher Certification program and have completed the required five hundred hours. I have more energy, vitality, and joy because of the changes I've made to create a simple life.

In my business, inner reflection forced me to be realistic about what energized me and what exhausted me. Always energized by speaking and training and the deep connection of one-on-one conversations, my love has always been helping people to be more successful and fulfilled in their lives. Sharing my knowledge and experience has been my gift to others, and that was important to maintain. Business can be super chaotic, and in the process of juggling all the hats we wear, we can forget what really brings us the most joy. I created a program called the Healthy Lifestyle Business.

To be a survivor and thrive in life, you will need to change, renew, empower, and transform your thinking, mindset, perception of yourself and life, your behaviors, habits, routines, choices, boundaries, and how you use your voice. It involves a life assessment—essentially deciphering what works and doesn't work for you personally.

After months of quiet time and reflection, I thought carefully about the aspects of life that helped me to change, renew myself, empower, and literally transform me. I focused on mindset, breath, movement, nutrition, heart and soul—what I call the six pillars of transformation and wellness for powerful living. Now I help others to do the same!

Life is marvelous! Love it… every single moment.

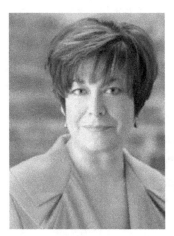

DEBORAH REYNOLDS *is an international speaker, bestselling author, and image expert. She helps high-achieving women hiding behind their current level of success to step out into who they are really meant to be so they can be healthier, happier, express their true gifts and brilliance, and make great money. Visit her website to download her free e-book,* Kick Start Your Business Image: 9 Keys to Get You Noticed, Known and Remembered.

www.deborahreynolds.com
www.aboutfaceforlife.com

REDEFINED COURAGE

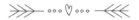

Nikki Speer

That morning in July of 2006 seems hazy now. This is how I remember it. I had an almost one-month-old little girl, Savannah, and a little five-year-old boy, Colin, at the time and my sweet Momma, Virginia, had just called to say she was headed over. I loved that we only lived a few miles apart because she's my best friend. I always welcomed her kind of company—you know, the kind you don't have to pick up, wipe down counters, or move the pile of clean clothes for. The best kind.

What I didn't welcome was the horrible news she brought with her that day. She spoke of cancer in her mammary ducts, the twelve to fourteen-hour tram flap surgery to remove the cancer and the treatment that would follow. What? Hadn't our family had enough of this? Wasn't two aunts and a grandmother diagnosed with cancer enough? God, what is going on? What could actually be the purpose of all this pain? To say that in these moments I became scared is an understatement.

2006 brought pain and healing, treatment and hope. Mom lost her hair and was very tired, but between working and resting, she gained strength and perspective. She found healing for herself and her relationship with my daddy.

We faced ongoing trials in the coming years: my husband, Gerrod, losing his job, getting pregnant with Emma seven months after Savannah was born (a blessing but stressful at the time), my husband going back to college to get his bachelors and masters, my preventative double mastectomy with spacers (my family history proved it was necessary), then an implant surgery because my right implant fell, recovery, depression, caring for my grandmother, Loretta, her passing away—and then, in 2011, my mom's five-year check-up. The news we had been waiting for was not the news we had expected to hear: "Your cancer has returned!" How could this be? We were absolutely devastated.

I couldn't handle the stress. I threw my hands up at God and said, "Nope, not doing this your way anymore." This led to living life like a selfish teenager. I was angry, miserable, and ungrateful; my heart was broken and I couldn't be thankful for the many blessings I had in front of me. I couldn't see clearly enough.

Aunt Katherine, my mom's youngest sister, passed away in December 2012, and the pain in my heart became even more unbearable. Breast cancer was the dirtiest word I had ever heard, and all the medicine, treatment, and pain that came with it was even worse.

Well, my mom is a fighter, so she went through her second surgery—a double mastectomy with spacers, followed by radiation treatment. She was scheduled to have implants, but something wasn't right. The incisions from the surgery weren't closing properly. Then red spots started to form on her breasts and torso, so there was another surgery and more chemotherapy.

I noticed that something amazing was happening, though

(when I wasn't focusing on myself). Mom was faithful to her God, smiling, and caring for others, and this was teaching me something. I didn't know what yet, but I somehow knew that after all this pain, there had to be a purpose. It was beginning to dawn on me that my own heart and relationships needed changing. Breast cancer was becoming my biggest teacher, and my mom was one of the strongest, most faith-filled people I knew.

In October 2015 all the chemotherapy was finished. Cancer had ravaged my mom's skin from the bottom of her neck to the bottom of her torso, and when it showed up in her spine, she officially was done with all the worldly treatment (that we are incredibly grateful and thankful for). I paid her a visit so we could spend quality time together. This time we weren't down the street in New York. Our little family had relocated to North Carolina.

It was so good to see her up and about when I arrived, and we planned to go to the mall and shop for clothes. We both love clothes and spending money, so it was the perfect plan! All the surgeries and treatment left Mom flat-chested, with a chemo belly, and lymphedema in her arms—she told me didn't feel like a woman at all! She walked out of the mall empty-handed. That's when I spoke these words: "Mom, someday I will design clothing for you to wear."

In the airport on my way home from New York, I felt a nudge from God to draw a shirt. Thinking this was crazy because I have no idea how to draw (my talents are spending money and talking, lol), I did it anyway. I drew a post-op shirt on the only thing I had in my purse, a sticky note. I drew the first thing a woman would need coming out of a breast surgery. She would have drains and limited mobility and would need clothing that encouraged healing during her recovery. When I returned home, I shared this idea with my husband and then started calling people and talking to everyone I knew about it.

A short two-and-a-half months later, I witnessed my precious mother take her last breath on December 5, 2015. Her body was now whole again, and she no longer was in pain.

This crazy idea I had to help my mom turned into samples, a business, a clothing line, a saving grace in my grief, and now a foundation to help others. Cancer has a way of redefining what you think courage is. To do things you've never done before, to live like you never have before, and to find hope where there seems to be none—in these moments you have Redefined Courage.

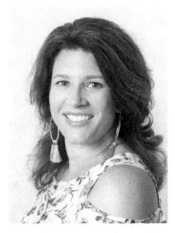

Nikki Speer *is married to the love of her life, Gerrod, and is the mother of Colin, Savannah, and Emma, her greatest treasures. Nikki is an author, speaker, avid walker, lover of people, and an aspiring minimalist. She is also the founder of Redefined Courage Foundation, gifting "HOPE" to women with breast cancer. This foundation was birthed from a promise to her late mother, Virginia. She and her family (including her daddy) reside in North Carolina.*

www.redefinedcourage.com

IT REALLY DOES TAKE A VILLAGE

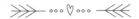

Karen Strauss

Barely glancing at me, the technician told me to go back to the waiting room as they needed to get more pictures of me. When you have had as many mammograms as I have, I knew what that meant.

I sat and waited, sat and waited some more. . . . I was petrified, anguished, paralyzed. I kept going up to the front desk and asking when they would call me back. I waited another thirty minutes, and finally I could not breathe—my adrenaline was pumping and I thought I was going to faint.

So I ran! Out of the double doors—out into the street where the sun was shining that warm July day. I ran to the bus to take me home so I could put my head under the covers, irrationally thinking that if the words weren't spoken, I wouldn't have the dreaded "c" word.

On the bus my cell phone kept ringing. When I got home, the phone was still ringing. I had several messages from the lab telling me it was urgent I go back.

I finally called them and scheduled my appointment for the next morning at 8:00 a.m. Next I called my best friend. She dropped everything and listened and then insisted that

71

she go with me the next day. It didn't hurt that she is a women's health provider and knows her way around a x-ray.

They confirmed that I had breast cancer. The bad news was that it had already started to spread outside the duct, but the cancer was really small and it had been caught early.

I will never forget the walk home, with my friend Susan holding my hand. She said, "You are going to be fine. It will be a rough journey for a while, but you will be just fine. You will come to see this as just a bump in the road.

Well, I am not going to lie. It felt like much more than a bump in the road during that long, dreadful year, but during that time I realized how many amazing friends and supporters I had.

The biopsy, endless meetings with surgeons, oncologists, my primary doctor . . . Susan was with me through all of it. I was so grateful to her; she was my advocate. She took notes; she could hear what the doctors were saying, while I could barely listen.

Finally we found the right team. I had the surgery—I needed a mastectomy. I woke up in the hospital to four worried faces trying to put on a brave front: my brother and sister-in-law, Susan, my cousin . . .

Everybody said at once, "It went great!" That was the beginning of my transformation, although I didn't know it yet.

You see, I had always been a very independent woman. Even when I was very young, I could always "do it myself." I didn't need anyone to help me; I was the one who people turned to when they needed to talk about their problems. I always saw needing help from someone as weak. I was the strong one. I was not going to be vulnerable—I would manage just fine!

Karen Strauss

I could take care of managing my business, my clients, my employees, my co-op, my house in the country, my dog—and now my cancer. This was just one more thing . . . right?

Well, I could not have been more wrong! I didn't realize what a big deal this was, and I needed to focus every bit of attention on getting well. From choosing the surgeon, the oncologist, getting second and third opinions to finally undergoing the surgery, enduring more endless tests, and setting up the chemo treatment. And then living with the effects of the chemo itself—the nausea, the fatigue, the memory loss . . .

Throughout this process, I don't know how I would have made it through without my family, good friends—surprisingly even those that weren't such good friends.

For instance, one person (now an Oscar winner for the movie *Birdland*!) who I knew from the dog park called me and offered to take my dog, Izzy, to the park anytime I wanted. I did not know him very well at that point, and his generous offer floored me.

Similar offers came. A woman in my building is a makeup artist, and when I had a swanky holiday party to attend, she offered to do my makeup—complete with false eyelashes!

And one night, when I decided it was time to cut the remaining hair on my head (a very emotional decision for me), my friend (whose husband works on Broadway) brought over one of her friends who cuts hair professionally for Broadway productions. They made it fun—we had champagne and hors d'oeuvres.

One neighbor, who I knew just to say hello to, came to

my apartment every night while I was going through chemo to check on me, see if I needed anything, and offer to walk Izzy. This was a lifesaver, since by then I was pretty wiped out and sometimes couldn't even make it off the couch, let alone get dressed in five layers, dress Izzy, and walk out in 10-degree weather so Izzy could do his business.

I could go on and on about the generosity and support offered to me by friends, family, and acquaintances who were ready and willing to do something, anything, to help me.

And for the first time in my life, I let them! Wow! What a feeling—I went from feeling guilty to feeling grateful and appreciative of the fact that so many people wanted to support and help me. All I had to do was say yes and give them a task.

So many people came to sit with me during the four hours each week I had my chemo treatment. My friends who thought they were stand-up comedians practiced on me, their captive audience. Some of my friends came to gossip, or spill their problems, or just discuss world events. I was SO grateful not to have to talk about "how I was feeling," or about my illness in general. It made the time fly by.

I have never forgotten this lesson. I no longer want to be a loner, to have to make decisions by myself, to not allow myself to be vulnerable. This has stood me in good stead to grow my business as well as become more intimate in my personal relationships.

I've learned that life is more fun when I let people in. I no longer feel the weight of the world on my shoulders. I know I have mentors, friends, advisors, and loved ones who will keep me grounded, supported, and constantly aware that I do not have to go through life alone.

It really does take a village—and I am deeply and profoundly grateful!

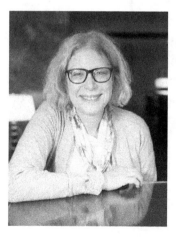

KAREN STRAUSS *has worked in publishing for more than thirty years and has held management and marketing positions at major publishing houses, including The Free Press, Crown, Random House, and Avon. Karen founded Hybrid Global Publishing in 2011 to help authors, speakers, and entrepreneurs get their message out by writing and publishing a book. She offers publishing, distribution, and marketing services for organizations and individual authors.*

www.hybridglobalpublishing.com

Our mission is to get *The Silver Lining of Cancer* into the hands of people across the world who need some inspiration, hope . . . and a guide to look for the silver lining at a scary time in their lives.

We hope you found at least one chapter that spoke to you . . . that was what you needed to read at that moment in time.

We'd love to hear from you!
Please join us on our Facebook Page
http://bit.ly/silverliningfb

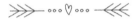

If you want to help us with our mission, we invite you to share this copy with family and friends, or purchase one as a gift for someone going through trying times. There is also an opportunity to purchase and donate books that will be delivered to support centers around the world. More details can be found on our Facebook page or on our website:

https://thesilverliningofcancer.com

"I alone cannot change the world, but I can cast a stone across the waters to create many ripples."
MOTHER TERESA

CPSIA information can be obtained
at www.ICGtesting.com
Printed in the USA
BVHW041928110419
545282BV00016B/254/P